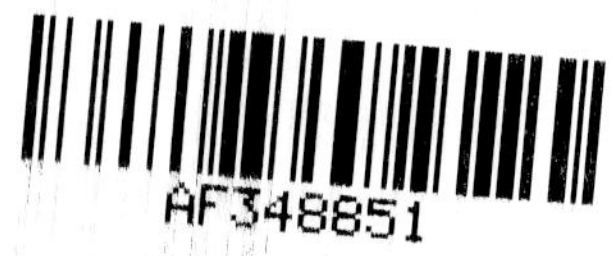

AF348851

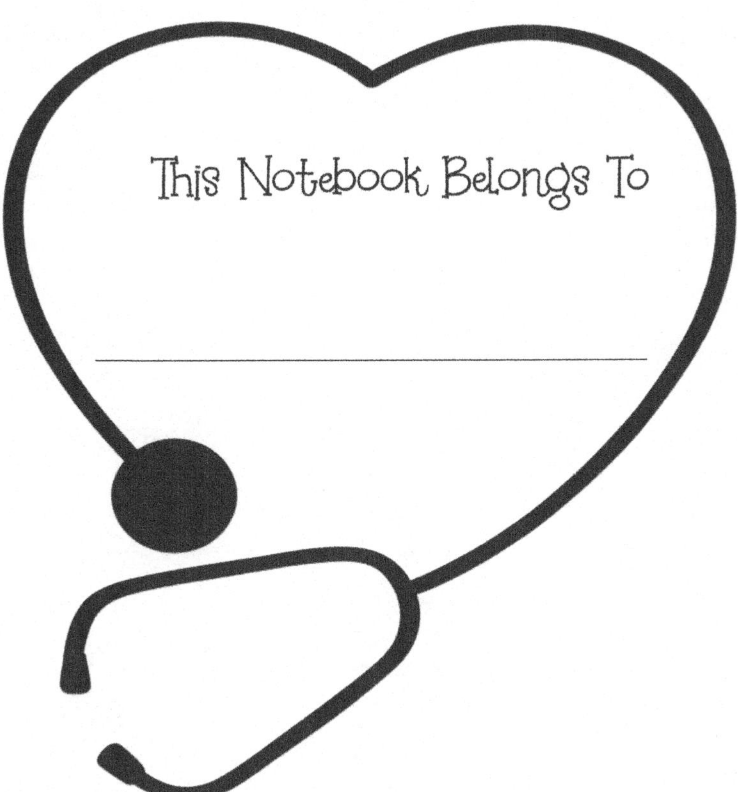

This Notebook Belongs To

Made in the USA
Monee, IL
07 July 2026

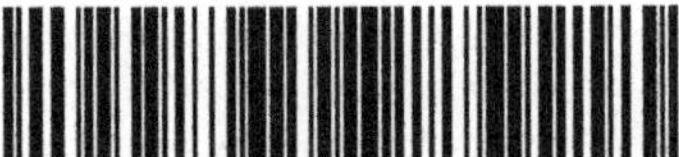

56552435R00070